I0481984

Autopsy of the NP

Dissecting the Nursing Profession
Piece by Piece

Nancy Congleton, RN

Autopsy of the NP: Dissecting the Nursing Profession Piece by Piece

© 2018 by Nancy Congleton, RN

Publisher: Nurse Nancy Press

DEDICATION

Dedicated to my grandfather Richard Hubbard,
and my husband David, for their *unwavering* support.

CONTENTS

INTRODUCTION

When I decided to become a nurse, I didn't have a clue. I wasn't aware of the educational options available to me, what nursing school was really like, or what to expect if I actually graduated and was thrown into the heart of the jungle!

Yes, my instructors did a fine job of lecturing, setting up skills labs, and testing us till our brains were nearly fried. But, they never enlightened us with the lowdown on this profession — the additional things you *really* need to know. Nor did I glean this invaluable information reading a bazillion textbooks or during my clinical rotations.

Did I ever catch on, get in the swing of things, and figure it out? Sure, I did! Once I was in the thick of it, with mounds of student loans to repay and burned bridges behind me. At that point though, what choice did I have?

To this day, I get a little frustrated with all the hype about being a nurse. Can the nursing profession be a great and wonderful occupation to be in? Absolutely! I just wish I'd been better prepared for it. And because of the nationwide nursing shortage, and therefore job security it provides, it's often portrayed as the golden goose by career advisors, who are NOT nurses.

So, if you're considering different career options and find yourself intrigued by what this profession can offer you – or you're already enrolled in a nursing program –

my time in the trenches will serve you well AND put you ahead of the game. I cover how to get started, unexpected realities you'll face, legal issues, and much more.

During my 15-plus years as a nurse, I've worked in a pediatric clinic, in the NICU (Newborn Intensive Care Unit) taking care of premature babies on ventilators, and in the ER juggling a variety of medical needs and assisting with codes, and my experience in case management opened my eyes to the political side of patient care.

If you want a book comprised only of touchy-feely-heartwarming nursing stories, this isn't it. If you're just interested in the pros and cons of being a nurse, you can Google that. But emotional highs never last, and a brief list is no match for personal experience acquired through blood, sweat, and tears!

When I started my journey to become a nurse, there were endless employment opportunities, and that remains true today. According to the Bureau of Labor Statistics Occupational Outlook Handbook, found online, "Employment of registered nurses is projected to grow 15 percent from 2016 to 2026, much faster than the average for all occupations; and the employment of licensed practical nurses is projected to grow 12 percent from 2016 to 2026, faster than the average for all occupations." Therefore, if you want to be a nurse, rest assured a job will be waiting for you. But is this what you *really* want?

In nursing school, you'll learn about drugs, disease,

and death, but there's more to it than that. And hats off to you if you've never missed an episode of *Grey's Anatomy* – but nope, they don't have it right either. Being a nurse isn't just about blood and guts, making out in supply closets, and poop!

Want to know the essential components of being a nurse? From the great to the frustrating to the absolutely need-to-know? Then why not go to the source and get the scoop, according to one!

Shall we begin?

Getting Started

CHAPTER 1

Educational options: Two pathways to choose from

I don't recall the day or whether it was spring or fall, but I do remember this: I'd had about all I could take, and from somewhere deep within me a voice declared, *Nancy, this just won't do!* My husband and I were both working full time, we lived in a small affordable home, our cars were NOT brand new, nor did they go "zoom-zoom." But the reality was this: We made enough money to cover our mortgage, vehicle payments, and utilities; groceries, gas, and everything else went on the credit card.

As one season gave way to another, the balance on our card multiplied like rabbits and my stress level soared. It became clear that if something didn't change we would soon find ourselves in a full-blown financial crisis. It was at this *exact* moment that my journey to becoming a nurse began, and I immediately sought answers to these questions: How long will I be in college for this, how much will it cost me, and approximately how much will I make? Seventeen years ago I found the answers to be encouraging, and they remain optimistic today.

In regards to time, right now you can be an LPN (licensed practical nurse) in as little as 12 months, with some programs lasting up to 18 months. Or, you can become a registered nurse with an associate degree. If you don't have any college credits, with this option you're looking at about three years, including basics and the core nursing program.

As for the cost, this can vary. LPNs go to a trade/ vocational school where the average is $10,000 to $15,000 nationally, with some being as low as $5,000. The Northeast Tech center located in my area was charging $5,400 in-state tuition for their one-year LPN program, as of May 2018.

Or, if you want to pursue an associate degree in nursing, you can attend a community college or a well-known university and stay local or have out-of-state living expenses. Your answers to these questions will ultimately determine how much this education will cost you, but an estimate from looking at multiple programs is an average of $35,000 and upwards for an associate degree in nursing.

My associate degree from Rogers State University in my hometown of Claremore, Oklahoma, cost approximately $8,000 over a decade ago. RSU no longer offers an associate degree in Nursing; it has been replaced with a 4-year BSN program. The approximate cost for in-state tuition for the BSN program is $39,892 which includes the prerequisite and core nursing classes, as of May 2018.

One of the great things about the nursing profession

is you can start with the minimum requirements to practice and later build on your education if you want to. My sister did this. She became an LPN, worked a couple of years, and then enrolled in an LPN to RN bridge program.

In regards to the average starting salary for a nurse, this depends on which state you live in and your area of practice. I encourage those interested to search online for their particular state and research different specialties (home health nurse, ER nurse, mental health nurse, etc.) for a ballpark amount.

Just to give you a general idea: In May 2016, the median annual wage for an LPN was $44,090 and for an RN it was $68,450, according to the Bureau of Labor Statistics Occupational Outlook Handbook, found online. This means half the nurses earned more than this amount and half earned less.

All in all, this is a pretty good deal. Want to jump in as quickly as possible? Then perhaps the LPN route is best for you. Or, if you can invest a little more time and money at the start, then consider going for your RN. Regardless of which path you choose or how long you're on it, let's be clear: As a nurse, it's not likely you'll ever be rollin' down the highway in a fully loaded Mercedes-Benz like a neurosurgeon might. But, you also won't be in college for approximately 14 years or have nightmares about brains. At least I hope not.

CHAPTER 2

Vaccines, background checks, and moments of delirium

I'll never forget one particular evening in my anatomy and physiology class. As soon as the clock revealed it was time to begin, our instructor announced that we'd be looking at urine under a microscope. Up to this point, our projects had involved dissecting pigs, sheep eyeballs, etc., so I half expected an old, rusty can of pig or sheep urine to appear before us – but no such thing occurred. Instead, she pulled out urine specimen cups (like the kind you get at the doctor's office) and informed us that we'd be providing our own sample for that evening's project. While the thought of playing with my own urine was utterly disgusting, for the first time in my life I was thankful for my tiny bladder and ability to pee on demand.

This particular memory will be forever stuck in my brain, but it is only a *glimpse* of this stage of my journey; therefore, let's start at the beginning. Before getting accepted into a nursing program, you'll need to complete your basics and nursing prerequisites. And yes, as part of this, you'll create your own memories of dissection and other squishy, gross things.

Next, apply for the nursing program that has caught your eye. But before doing that – and regardless of which program you enroll in (LPN or RN) – you need to ask the enrollment department about their NCLEX pass rate. This is the state test you take after you've completed a nursing program in order to receive your nursing license. While it is the student's responsibility to study and learn the material, the institution needs to lecture and test on the most prevalent information to prepare the student for the NCLEX exam and the profession itself. So if a nursing program has a decent pass rate – 85 percent or higher – it's a good sign they're staying current on nursing practices and teaching valuable content.

Following acceptance into a nursing program, they'll run a background check since you'll be going into hospitals, around sick patients, and near controlled substances. So if you've ever done time for severing someone's brake lines, or redistributing their money to an offshore account for safekeeping, then it would be wise to call and discuss this with the nursing program you wish to attend AND the Board of Nursing, before you do anything else.

You'll also be required to get some vaccinations. You'll need to get a TB (tuberculin) skin test. Your tetanus vaccine will need to be up to date. If you've had chicken pox, you won't need the varicella vaccine; if you haven't had it, you will. You'll be required to get the MMR (measles, mumps & rubella) vaccine and a hepatitis B series, which consists of three shots.

There are some exceptions to these vaccinations. For example, if you've already received the hepatitis B series and have a blood test showing your titers/immunities are high, then you won't need to get them again. For complete guidelines and any questions, inquire with the nursing enrollment department.

Now, every nursing program has its own structure, but you'll be learning the same things. Biology, anatomy and physiology, and pharmacology are a few of the basic classes. Next, there are different areas of nursing, such as maternal and newborn, pediatrics, medical-surgical, and emergency nursing. Again, these are just a few, but with mountains of information to cover, gear up to read and study more than ever and feel free to say goodbye to any and all hobbies for the foreseeable future.

On your clinical days (following another nurse and helping take care of patients) you'll rise at the crack of dawn, and facilities do limit how many nursing students can be onsite at the same time. Therefore, you don't always get to do your clinical rotations at the nearest facility from your home. I had some that were an hour away, and I had to be there by 6:30 a.m.

In regards to your clinical days, they're meant to be a hands-on learning opportunity, and yet many students focus on looking through charts instead of grasping every chance to give a shot, start an IV, or witness a procedure.

Most nurses are so busy they don't have time to encourage you to participate, so be watchful for these learning opportunities and step forward when they arise.

To be honest, though, your clinical rotations won't *fully* prepare you to be a nurse. I compare this to people who think they know how to be a parent because they watched their friends' kids over the weekend; it's just not the same. But if you make the most of your clinical experience, you'll acclimate more easily when you are a nurse.

Next, I'll share with you a complication of nursing school that may seem unlikely, and I hope it is for you. Occasionally, when people begin making positive changes in their life — whether in the pursuit of a nursing degree or any advancement — it can make those around them uncomfortable. Here are two reasons for this: They see you overcoming roadblocks to have a better life, and it reminds them of the obstacles overtaking theirs. Or, they themselves are successful and do not want everyone else joining this elite club. This discomfort can present itself as tension, moodiness, or slightly negative questions or comments regarding what you are trying to accomplish.

My nursing professors had seen this issue manifest many times before and therefore addressed it the first week of school. I did not experience this while in the nursing program, but after I passed state boards I got major pushback from someone. If this happens to you, don't get caught off guard or confront the person. Keep your eyes on the prize and take care of business.

Also, try not to panic too much regarding weight gain, bouts of crying, or brief moments of insanity. At some point, it happens to all of us. My turn came one evening after studying for hours and then crashing on the couch. My sweet husband was working nights at the time and thought it'd be a *wonderful* idea to call and check on me. While still asleep I somehow managed to grab the phone, but in my study-induced delirium I answered it shouting, "I gave you your Tylenol already!"

What happened to our marriage? It's still on track and he adores me more than ever. No, seriously, he does.

Hours of Operation and Varying Nursing Environments

CHAPTER 3

Oh, the scheduling options you'll have!

I'll confess something to you. I loathe the Monday – Friday, 8 to 5 type schedule. I've done it, and not only did I completely disdain it, I felt like a mindless drone: getting up at the same time five days in a row, driving to the same place, doing the same work with the same people (no offense, people). But throw a 12-hour shift at me and it's a different story. I know my day's going to be long, but that's ok. I'm strapped in and ready to do my time because I won't be doing it five days in a row.

Now, you might be reading this and thinking, *No way do I want 12-hour shifts!* That's OK; the nursing profession provides so many opportunities to work that you can find a time frame that suits you best. In no particular order, here are some options for you to think about.

As a full-time home health nurse, this is usually a Monday – Friday position and your start time can vary. If you have a patient who rises early, you could see them at 7 a.m. and possibly be finished by 4 p.m. Or, if you have patients who prefer to be seen in the evenings, you could start your day later. It all depends on your caseload, patient availability, and distance between patients. Keep in mind, though, that some home health companies have their nurses rotate after-hours on-call and cover weekends.

If you're interested in working as a hospice nurse, your schedule will be similar to that of a home health nurse, with the exception that when a patient is in the active process of dying, hospice nurses normally provide round-the-clock care for the patient and the family. During this time hospice nurses do switch out at certain intervals, but this can cause you to work beyond your normal scheduled hours.

Do you really want off evenings, weekends and holidays? Then working as a school nurse, in a doctor's office, at a health department, or for a medical insurance company will be your best options; they're usually Monday – Friday, 8 to 5.

However, if you want to be a school nurse, know that this usually requires a bachelor's degree. According to a relative of mine who worked as a school nurse, you can have an associate degree in nursing with a bachelor's in something else, but you need to have a bachelor's, or be actively working on it.

In regards to hospitals, most have adapted to 12-hour shifts for nursing staff, but there are several departments that run off 8-hour schedules. First, I'll talk about some of the 12-hour shifts: The standard shifts are 7 a.m. to 7 p.m. and 7 p.m. to 7 a.m. These are typical of medical-surgical floors, intensive care units, and pediatrics, to name a few.

Most ERs work with your basic 7 to 7 start times, and 10 a.m. to 10 p.m., 3 p.m. to 3 a.m., or a similar variation. ERs try to provide the most coverage during the busiest times, and scheduling like this works well for them.

As an OR (operating room) nurse, you'll have an earlier start time (around 6 a.m.), but you're usually finished around 3 p.m. If you're fulltime, this is a Monday – Friday schedule with rotating on-call.

If you work in a cardiac cath lab, you'll have a Monday – Friday schedule with a time frame of 6 a.m. to 3 p.m., 7 a.m. to 4 p.m., or something close to it.

If you work in risk management or as a quality assurance nurse, you're looking at Monday – Friday, 8 to 5.

Another nursing department within a hospital that works days is case management. This is sometimes an 8 a.m. to 4:30 p.m. position, or it can be 7 a.m. to 3:30 p.m. When I worked in case management, my hours were 7 a.m. to 3:30 p.m., and I rotated on-call and worked every third weekend. However, there were many times when situations developed that caused me to work over or come in while on-call to address immediate issues.

One more option for 8-hour shifts is working for an inpatient behavioral health facility. Their schedules are usually 7 a.m. to 3 p.m., 3 p.m. to 11 p.m., and 11 p.m. to 7 a.m., with a 30-minute allowance to give report to the next oncoming shift. These facilities are open 24/7 so rotating weekends is usually required.

If you don't mind working weekends (or would prefer them), there are some hospitals that offer 'weekend option' positions. You work 12-hour shifts every weekend and pick up either a Monday or Friday. These positions usually compensate very well, and there are advantages to having a set schedule.

In addition to those already mentioned, nurses also work for nursing homes, the American Red Cross, urgent care clinics (which vary in hours of operation), and dialysis clinics, as well as private-duty nursing with hours according to the patient's needs. Furthermore, there are some companies that employ nurses on-site to assess sick employees and/or on-the-job injuries.

This is a good overall view of most of the nursing schedules available and their accompanying areas, but no doubt there'll be some I missed. I hope what jumps out at you is this: As a nurse you can work days, evenings, nights, 12-hour shifts, 8-hour shifts, weekends or Monday – Friday. With so many opportunities to work, nurses simply have no excuse not to!

CHAPTER 4

From ER to home health and beyond:
Which area will suit you best?

I'd just started my shift one day and had other things needing my attention, but I simply *had* to see it. As I approached the grungy bucket just inside the patient's room, my heart quickened. I leaned forward, having been told the snake was dead but still half expecting it to strike. By the looks of it, I wasn't convinced it wouldn't! The poisonous snakes around my house are hacked to pieces, yet the one before me remained intact.

Although this is not the only ER escapade I've experienced. In addition to snakes in buckets, I've been handed fingers over ice in cups and seen the aftermath of toes colliding with lawnmowers. There's no set pattern or criteria for the ER, so *anything* is possible.

If this type of working environment is not your cup of tea, no problem! One of the things I LOVE about this profession is that it offers something for everyone. If I tried to cover *every* nursing specialty in detail, this chapter would go on forever, so here's a crash course on some of your options.

If you're not too keen on surprises and prefer consistency, newborn nursery might be worth considering. You'll do the initial newborn assessment, which includes measurements, vitamin K injection, erythromycin ointment in the babies' eyes and determine their Apgar score (a score based on the infant's heart rate, respiratory effort, muscle tone, reflex irritability, and color after delivery). Then each shift will do a basic assessment, and you'll monitor feeding, bathing, vital signs, and diaper changes, as well as see the baby back and forth to the parents' room. Occasionally, there'll be an undetected medical complication that arises, but most of the time the work is routine and consistent.

If you work on a medical-surgical floor, you might have a patient with pneumonia, a post-hysterectomy patient, and so on. As the name suggests, some of your patients will have a medical issue and some will be recovering from surgery.

Think you'd enjoy taking care of children? You could work in pediatric home health (taking care of medically fragile infants and children), a pediatric urgent care clinic, or a pediatrician's office. If you want to take care of children in a hospital setting, you could work on a pediatric floor, in pediatric ICU, or in pediatric oncology.

Love mental health? There are mental health facilities that provide care 24/7 and meet the needs of all ages, from adolescence to geriatrics; or you could do follow-up care as a psychiatric home health nurse. Also, there are nursing homes that specialize in the care of dementia, and others that provide extensive rehabilitation after a stroke or a fall.

Some additional options are surgery or pre-op. For all of you who are antisocial, in these departments you don't have as much contact with patients compared to other areas.

Another option is a cardiac unit, or ICU step-down (a unit where patients are not critical enough to warrant intensive care but still too sick to be on a medical-surgical floor). Or you could work in adult home health (which can include patients released from the hospital but still recovering from an illness or post-surgery patients), in hospice (end-of-life care), as a school nurse, in a doctor's office, for the health department, or you could review cases for an insurance company.

Once you find your niche, gain some experience, and feel comfortable, you could work as an agency or travel nurse. As an agency nurse, you work for a nursing agency that provides nurses for other facilities, as well as home health and hospice companies. There are several great things about this. For one, you're basically an independent subcontractor, so you're never forced to work any particular shift. This may at times limit the shifts you have, but you do have a choice. You will also make more money per hour as an agency nurse.

As a travel nurse, you have the potential to make even *more* money. You could take an assignment in your own state or travel to another one. You're paid by the hour, plus you're given an allotment for living expenses as well. With some travel assignments you're offered a bonus, and some of these are large if you commit to an extended contract.

With all the different areas in nursing to choose from, you can find what works with *your* personality. Do you like fast, furious, bizarre, and different? ER could be your perfect fit. Like constantly meeting new faces but not taking care of them all day? Then pre-op, post-op, or a clinic might interest you. Are you detail-oriented, want to focus on one patient at a time, and don't like 12-hour shifts? Consider working as a home health nurse. Good with fluctuating emotions and not afraid of someone clasping your hand in a death grip? Labor and delivery might be your thing. I could continue, but I'll stop.

Bottom line? Your *beginning* options as a nurse are limitless, and if you decide at some point you want to advance in this profession, you've got multiple avenues. You can build on your education and become a nurse practitioner, a nurse anesthetist, or a nursing instructor – and these are just a few of your choices!

My personal recommendation is this: Mix it up. Challenge yourself. Diversify! Learn an area really well and stay there for a while. But if you become bored, static, or need a change of scenery, do something different within the profession. It's what I did, because as a nurse you're never stuck in the same loop, unless you want to be.

Nursing Attire and Body Mechanics

CHAPTER 5

It's not about fashion, y'all!

Prior to becoming a nurse I worked for a title and abstract company Monday through Friday. Our attire wasn't business casual, but I'd say one step below that. At the same time, my husband and I had bought our first house and were acclimating to new expenses, like a lawnmower. Gone were the days of our two-story, maintenance-free apartment; hello mortgage and grass. So buying new clothes for my five-day-a-week job wasn't ideal.

I still remember the dread of looking through my closet and thinking, *What am I going to wear? What did I wear last?* And then came the strategizing. *I wore that blouse with this skirt last Friday, so now I'll wear it with these pants.* And don't even get me started on the mornings I awoke to find I'd mysteriously gained weight overnight. Somehow, I made it work for two and a half years, but not without much frustration and a lot of planning.

When I became a nurse, my work-wardrobe crisis dissipated. I found good quality scrub sets for $40 and quality shoes for about the same. No more worrying about what I wore first or last and forget fretting over the right belt, shoes, or accessories. I could finally just throw on a potato sack and head to the factory to do my time.

However, during my stent in this profession, I've noticed that other nurses do NOT share my opinion. You see, while scrubs are indeed affordable, easy to care for and long-lasting – flattering they are not!

Many times, I've seen nurses attempt to compensate for this. They will wear tops so tight there's no *way* they can adequately breathe. Or, their pants will be at least one size too small. Sometimes, nurses will adjust in other ways, like wearing an excessive amount of bracelets or long, dangly earrings. I don't follow this either. When you're running in and out of homes doing home-health visits or rounding a busy corridor at a hospital, who wants to get slapped in the face by long, dangly earrings? Who knows, maybe these nurses don't run.

Bottom line? The nursing profession isn't meant to be glamorous. You're not dressing for the Grammys and nobody cares what the cool nurse is wearing. Should you fix your hair, iron your scrubs, and splash on a bit of make-up? Of course! You're a professional, so look like one. But, just take my word that when you're bent over a patient trying to start an IV or assisting the doctor with a procedure – accentuating your hips or your thighs or anything else you might have in mind *won't* be a priority.

CHAPTER 6

You won't sit or stand all day, but you might break your back!

Many years ago I worked in a department store. It was grueling but not necessarily because of the job. It wasn't hard straightening clothes and putting up sale signs; it was standing on my feet all day with no place to sit. By the time the day was over, I was exhausted and my back, calves, and feet were throbbing.

I also once worked as a secretary for a small real estate business. I sat at a desk, answered phones, labeled files, and sorted mail. Guess what? That was exhausting as well!

Eventually I figured out the body needs a little bit of everything. We need to stand, bend, turn, move, sit, rest, and exert. If we're sitting most of the time, we'll get tight muscles, which can lead to feeling stiff, or we'll get sleepy. But, if most of our work is done while standing, we'll have pain – usually in the back, legs, and feet.

So the best option is to have a balance of rest and movement, and *most* nursing positions provide this. For example, if you work at a doctor's office, you'll look through electronic medical records and return phone calls, but you'll also be up administering needed injections and assisting with any in-office procedures. As a home health nurse, you'll gather any needed supplies from the main office and then set out to see your patients, where you'll check vital signs, set up their medications, change any wound dressings they have, and draw blood from time to time. And, of course, if you work in a hospital or a clinic, you'll be in and out of patients' rooms and then sit down to complete your charting.

Now, maybe you're like me and find this variety of movement to be very appealing. That's great, but we need to look at the other side of this: In the nursing profession we frequently face unpredictable and awkward situations that put our bodies at great risk for injury.

For example, one day while working in the ER, my co-workers and I heard someone laying on their car's horn. Then immediately thereafter, we got a call from one of the ER clerks informing us that a body had just been dumped out in the ER circle drive.

What did we do? We grabbed a stretcher, ran to where the body was, and deadlifted the person – who was obviously now our responsibility – onto the stretcher. *Did all of us who lifted this person risk injuring our necks and backs?* Absolutely, but our approved lift equipment doesn't reach the floor, and we needed to start CPR immediately.

Here's another situation I have witnessed variations of: A patient with no activity restrictions but still recovering from surgery gets up to go to the bathroom and faints.

In addition to being unconscious, the patient could've hit his head on the way down and been bleeding as well, or possibly have lost control of his bowel or bladder. So now you're in a situation where you're expected to physically lift this patient off the floor as fast as possible – and you could be exposed to blood or bodily fluids at the same time.

I've also seen patients come to the ER with chest pain and drop in the lobby with a heart attack. There are some people who feel the effects of pain meds more than others and when they stand get dizzy and fall. This actually happened to my husband when he got Dilaudid for the first time.

Most people don't realize it, but these situations happen to nurses, and other medical personnel, all the time. This is also NOT isolated to hospital nursing. If you work for a clinic or as a school nurse, someone could faint or have a seizure, putting you in a lifting or injury-prone situation. If you work for home health or hospice, you might have to turn a patient or help him get out of bed or to the bathroom, all of which involve lifting. If there are family members present, they may be advanced in years and not able to help you.

Bottom line? The nursing profession in general is hard on the body: long hours, stressful situations, and required lifting. And then factor in all the awkward, spontaneous events that can and do happen – well, that's a strong recipe for disaster, and apparently disaster strikes often. According to surveys done by the Department of Labor's Bureau of Labor Statistics, there are more than 35,000 back and other injuries among nursing employees every year, severe enough that they have to miss work.

And what happens when a nurse is injured? At some facilities a drug screen is done immediately. (Personally, I find this more than reasonable. If an injury is related to drugs or alcohol, the company should NOT be held responsible. However, if you're a straight shooter, this can be insulting.) Next, the injured employee is sent to a work compensation doctor, many of whom could care less about them and downplay their injury regardless of what their tests show.

What's the final outcome for injured nurses? Far too many end up requiring surgery, addicted to pain pills, or on permanent or modified work restrictions.

One more thing: I find it interesting that some construction workers (who are usually big, strong men) are prevented from lifting more than 35 pounds while on the job. But if a nurse has a patient who's 125 pounds or less, we consider them lightweight.

Unexpected Realities

CHAPTER 7

Nursing school doesn't cover everything
you need to know.

It's been a while since I've purchased a brand-new vehicle, and I'm not looking forward to doing it again. Yes, the new-car smell is charming, but the valley of deception leading up to it is certainly not, for this is how it usually goes down: You look at the car, take it for a spin, check out the price on the windshield, and then go inside to do "the paperwork".

Four hours later, what you thought was a $20,000 car is now $25,000. And when you question the trustworthy salesman before you, he educates you that the price on the windshield doesn't cover the heated-seat feature, tires, or gas in the tank!

I experienced this same frustration on my journey to becoming a nurse. After all, the purpose of going to nursing school is that you *learn* how to be a nurse, right? Well, sort of. My professors explained it like this: We would learn the basics of nursing and cover as much as possible from all the nursing categories: pediatrics, emergency nursing, medical-surgical, mental health, maternal, newborn, and gerontology. But, if we tried to read, lecture, and test on everything in these areas, we'd be in school forever.

On one hand, this greatly reduced the length of time before I could practice. On the other hand, while I was credentialed as a nurse, I was not yet fully equipped. Furthermore, the nursing profession yields additional complexities. Not only is all the information in each area NOT covered, it is impossible to prepare students for the different scenarios that occur. For example, in nursing school you're taught about congestive heart failure, which includes signs and symptoms, prescribed medications, activity intolerances, and diet modifications. You're also taught the same things for diabetes.

So if you have a patient with congestive heart failure, there are things you watch for and address. If you have a patient with diabetes, there are things you watch for and address. But what if you have a patient with congestive heart failure AND diabetes? You now have two separate disease processes, each with its own standard of care yet intersecting in the same patient. Therefore, you must manage this patient's care with both pathways in mind.

Another scenario is this: You work in the ER and a patient comes in with a stab wound to the upper abdomen. The patient's friends tell you he was also ingesting alcohol and taking narcotics prior to that. So what you really have is a stab wound that could involve a vital organ and possible impending respiratory depression related to the combination of alcohol and narcotics.

One more example, this time from a different setting: As a home health nurse you arrive at your patient's house anticipating a wound care visit with a dressing change. Instead, you discover she's been vomiting for the last two days. Your original focus was just a dressing change, but inadequate nutrition will impede a wound from healing – so you must address the vomiting.

Generally speaking, in nursing school you learn one disease process at a time. One procedure or surgery at a time. One complication at a time. But more often than not, there are multiple things to consider with each patient. This, coupled with not covering everything from each area, can sometimes lead to much frustration and anxiety for a new nurse, or even an old one!

CHAPTER 8

I didn't know hospital nursing came with all that...

Every year my mom, sister, and I have a girl's day out shopping for our birthdays, and at some point find ourselves at the mall food court. We've burned some calories and need to refuel, and while the food court is NOT considered fine dining, it does provide an assortment of options that never fail to satisfy!

To me, a hospital is like a mall food court for nurses. You have one vast central location with varying environments, age groups, and a multitude of medical needs. From ER to newborn nursery, most nurses can find exactly what they're craving. However, while this buffet of choices seems appealing, don't be fooled by eye-candy; there's another side of the coin I'd like to share with you.

First off, I'll point out something obvious that's taken for granted. Hospitals do business 24/7, which means in order for them to run efficiently, schedules cannot be changed at the eleventh hour. Therefore, if your spouse plans a surprise Valentine weekend at your favorite destination, you are not guaranteed to get the time off. If you're scheduled to work, you'll either work or find another nurse to work for you, if your manager allows that.

Now when it comes to Thanksgiving, you could request off six months in advance, but don't be surprised if you work while Jenny Ann gets the day off. And, no doubt, you'll want to corner your manager and highlight that Jenny Ann is divorced, has no children, and lives with eight cats – but this won't be relevant. For if everyone wants Thanksgiving off, some will have to sacrifice their plans and work it.

To be honest, November and December are the worst months to be a hospital nurse. Once the holiday schedule gets posted the claws come out, and they are sharp! Almost everyone has a reason why they should get preferential treatment. *I have seniority in the department. But I've been a nurse longer than you. Hey, I have three children and you only have two!* And don't be shocked when someone plans their conception or schedules surgery in such a way as to be off work during these two months.

Hospitals also take NO consideration for the weather. While some jobs will let you take a personal day or remote in from home, for most nursing positions this is not an option and you'll be expected to find a way in – even if that means totaling your car on the way and presenting with frostbite.

In regards to weekends, almost every nursing department in a hospital works weekends. The surgery department doesn't schedule surgeries on the weekend, but they rotate on-call for any emergent surgeries needed over the weekend or after normal hours. The rest of the departments work weekends. Typically, you rotate weekends and just work every other one.

When deciding whether to work days versus nights in a hospital, there are some notable differences worth mentioning. For one, day shift is usually very hectic. In addition to regular admits, most surgeries are scheduled during the day, whether it's open heart surgery, cataract surgery, or a planned C-section. Therefore, day shift usually receives more admits than night shift.

Also during the day, the administrative staff is on-site. Sometimes they make rounds through the departments and ask how everyone's doing. However, if they see anything concerning – in regards to a patient, family member, staff, or even equipment – they will on occasion stop you and address it. Be prepared to have an answer.

Regarding night shift, you can get admits from the ER, take on emergency surgeries, and of course babies can arrive at any time. But night shift does have a more relaxed, quiet feel to it. All the scheduled surgeries are usually done, there are no meetings taking place, only the core hospital staff is present, and usually patients want to rest and go to sleep.

The drawback is this: If something goes wrong on night shift, you don't have the resources and support that are available during the day. Some hospitals do employ nurse 'house supervisors' to help at night, but administration is gone, the managers are gone, and you don't have as many physicians on-site.

Another situation to be aware of if you work in a hospital is 'forced floating.' Now, some nurses get established in their home department and then cross-train to other areas. This allows them to pick up additional shifts, learn something new, and get paid extra every time they float out of their home department.

But forced floating is different. This happens when a department doesn't have enough patients for the amount of nurses that are scheduled to work that shift. So, you are forced to float to another area in the hospital that has MORE patients than the nurses currently scheduled.

Forced floating can cause a lot of stress on staff. Not only is it stressful for the nurse being floated, but also for the department the nurse is floated to. In the midst of their work, they need to provide a quick orientation for someone unfamiliar with their department. This can include everything from where the supplies are to that unit's policies and procedures.

Most facilities try to be somewhat reasonable about this. For example, if you work in newborn nursery, it's not likely you'll be floated to the ER. But, you might get floated to pediatrics, and that's different than newborn nursery. As a new nurse, and definitely while on orientation, you won't get floated to another area. But once the hospital views you as an established nurse, you'll be fair game!

In addition to forced floating, sometimes you'll be forced to 'flex off' a shift if the hospital doesn't have enough patients for everyone scheduled. This can happen to any department at any time but occurs more in summer months when flu and pneumonia are not as prevalent. If you need a full paycheck and have PTO available, you can use it. Yes, you'd probably want to save that PTO for a vacation, but it is what it is.

If at this point you still feel bewitched by the idea of hospital nursing with all those cool departments to choose from, then know this: Sometimes it takes trying different things before discovering your perfect fit. There's nothing wrong with this, but know that most hospitals want you to stay in a department for six months prior to transferring to another one. So if you start off in pediatrics but find it breaks your heart to stick children with needles, well, more than likely you'll be sticking it out. No pun intended.

CHAPTER 9

By the way, you're supposed to know it all!

Every time I hear the phrase, *Hey, you're a nurse!* it's like a nuclear power plant just began its countdown to complete and utter annihilation. I have no idea from which area of nursing their questions will fire from, and my brain begins to power down. Will they be seeking answers in regards to cardiac nursing, pediatric nursing, surgical nursing, trauma nursing... who knows! And yet, this is the expectation from the public, your family, and friends – that YOU (the nurse) should know everything. On one hand, it's a compliment for them to think of nurses as having all the answers, but it's unrealistic and annoying.

Consider this – doctors go to medical school and then choose the area they want to specialize in: pediatrics, cardiology, oncology, etc. They're not an expert in all things. That's why physicians give referrals to patients when they need a specialist and consult with other physicians in their same field when they have a difficult case.

If you asked a dermatologist what the most life-threatening complications of pregnancy are, he probably wouldn't have those answers handy. If you questioned a family medicine physician about the process of cardio-thoracic surgery, more than likely she wouldn't know all the details.

This same theory applies to nurses. As I've previously mentioned, we attend nursing school, get a general knowledge base, and decide which area of nursing to work in, then (hopefully) learn as much as possible in *that* area.

Furthermore, the medical field is ever changing. What was the recommended treatment for xyz eight months ago will not necessarily be the advised treatment today. In addition, we live in the age of Internet searches, so even if you're certain you're giving accurate information in hopes of helping someone, there's the potential for an article, physician, or clinical study found online that conflicts with the info you give.

Also, some people know just enough about a medical topic or situation to be contentious. In reality, they know a little but present as though they know a lot and will argue with you to no end. Bless their little hearts.

Not only during my years as a nurse have I occasionally disappointed others, but to be perfectly honest, I also disappoint myself from time to time. Such a moment occurred one evening when I was appointed charge nurse on a psychiatric floor.

At first I had no cause for alarm, for I'd been charge nurse many times before, in that department and others. But when I witnessed something entirely disgusting and vomited on the floor, the toilet, and myself, it became quite embarrassing to yell down the hall for help.

What made it even worse was that my dinner that evening consisted of tomatoes and strawberries. Therefore, when my supportive staff came to my rescue, it appeared I was in the midst of a bloody massacre.

As a nurse, even though you can't and won't know everything, or handle every situation with dignity, you will have many opportunities to help those who do fall into your field of expertise. So if your neighbor, in-laws, or anyone else makes you feel stupid for not having all the answers, just smile politely, be a tad naughty, and tell them you've been winging it!

Trying Relationships and My Tips for Surviving Them

CHAPTER 10

It's hit and miss with patients!

I'd just received an ambulance patient one day and rushed into the room to assess her, but the second she laid eyes on me she shouted, "You can't be my nurse, you're just a little girl!" I immediately attempted to quell her fears with the knowledge that I was actually in my thirties and had been practicing for a while, but she would have nothing of it.

I also encountered a patient who after glancing at the stethoscope around my neck said, "Do you have a license for that?" I showed her my RN identification; she informed me that at the Ne-Mar Shopping Center you can buy any certificate you want!

So if you want to know the scoop on patients, here it is: Some patients will think you're the best nurse ever (even when you're not) and want to squeeze you like a Care Bear. Others will stare at you like you're Captain Stupid who's just returned from Mars three years past the landing date. But whether patients love you, hate you, or just don't know what to make of you – here are my tips for making the best of it!

Embrace the love. When tiny patients draw me pictures, I let my guard down and my heart soar. When elderly patients stroke my hair as their heading out the door, I smile sweetly. I've even had patients ask me for a hug, and I open wide my arms. There are plenty of other patients who show me their claws, so if a patient wants to love on me (within reason of course) I just soak it up like rays of sunshine.

Don't take things personally. Being a patient – at the mercy of doctors and nurses – is a vulnerable place to be. Patients are often scared, hurting, and frustrated, and feel as if they don't have a voice. So try not to be too self-absorbed; on many occasions it's not actually about you.

Stick to the facts. When you have a grumpy patient who's trying to bully you into doing something you shouldn't, use the words 'policy,' 'procedure,' 'protocol,' and/or 'medical guidelines.' Here's how you do it: *I'm sorry, sir, that you want two weeks off work for a sinus infection, but it's our policy to write work notes for only the amount of time the physician feels is necessary.*

Or, *I'm sorry, ma'am. I have indeed heard your request for pain pills, sleeping pills, and the strongest muscle relaxer available, but it's against medical guidelines to prescribe patients a cocktail of drugs that could lead to respiratory depression and death.*

Always tell the truth. If a patient asks you a question and you honestly don't know the answer, just say something like, *Off the top of my head I'm not sure, but I'll find out and be right back!* Or, if a patient asks you a question and you DO know the answer, be honest about that as well. I once walked into a room with a steroid injection for a patient. He looked at me hesitantly and said, "Are you any good at those?" To which I honestly replied, "I don't know, but I guess you're about to find out."

CHAPTER 11

Being in charge ain't a picnic.

One day in the midst of a conversation with a coworker (whom I was in charge of) I was referred to as 'fiddle-britches.' Now, my initial inclination was that this was NOT meant in an endearing way. Nonetheless, before becoming all-judgy, I thought I'd at least throw it at Google and see what it came up with.

There was certainly info to be found on the word 'fiddle' and the word 'britches,' but nothing whatsoever to guide me in the meaning of 'fiddle-britches.' My final thought (since this particular person had balked at my authority before) was that this wasn't spoken with the intention of, *You're so adorable for accomplishing so much at such a young age.*

Truth be told, I don't feel that I've accomplished all that much. And when I entered nursing school, the furthest thing from my mind was that in addition to being responsible for patient care, I'd one day be in charge of those I worked with. And yet, I wasn't licensed very long before finding myself in these situations.

So what do I do when I find myself in charge of nurse aids, nurse techs, medical assistants, etc. (with many being older than me)? Well, I do a couple of things depending on the situation, and here they are.

Set the tone. The first thing I do is take a long, hard look at myself. Am I the embodiment of what I expect from my coworkers? If not, then I'm missing the mark and it's time to get *myself* back on point!

Bull in the china shop. If something's unfolding (or about to unfold) that could negatively affect patient care or their final outcome, then I show my horns. Because, if something goes seriously wrong (that I could've prevented) while I'm in charge, it's on MY license, so you better believe I'm going to protect it.

Polite but firm. I believe in giving people a chance to do what they KNOW they need to do. But, if they don't *eventually* do their job, take care of patients, and support the team – I will call them out and *ask* them to do it. I will do it politely, I will say *please and thank you*, but I will do it!

Take one for the team. Occasionally, those I'm in charge of feel they absolutely must mouth off to me, or prove I'm wrong about something (and sometimes I am), or insult me in some way; there are moments when I just let this slide. Just because you're the boss doesn't mean you need to cram it down people's throats all the time.

Pray! When I absolutely can't get traction or unity with a subordinate, I pray.

Report to a higher authority. Negative patient outcomes are unacceptable, as is losing my license. If I can't resolve an issue with steps one through five – there's only one thing left!

CHAPTER 12

They're called mean nurses, and they are real!

I crossed paths one day with a friend I hadn't seen in a while, and in the process of catching up she asked what I was up to. So I eagerly divulged I was in nursing school, but her countenance quickly changed and she replied without hesitation, "Nurses eat their young, Nancy."

Now, I couldn't help erupting in laughter, but my friend wasn't laughing at all and followed her initial comment with, "Seriously, they can be mean." I remember later thinking it was strange for her to say such things when she didn't work in the medical profession. How on earth could she know for certain that some nurses are mean? However, once I found myself in the trenches, my friend's warning came back to me, and over the years I've learned she wasn't being facetious; nurses do indeed eat their young.

So what do I mean when I say 'nurses eat their young'? Well, here are some examples for us to look at. For one, a mean nurse can frequently and deliberately give you a hard assignment. I'll explain. All patients are not created equal. Some are alert, oriented, and fairly healthy;

others are confused, bedfast, and take ten different medications. Which of these two patients are going to be easier to take care of? Now, what if you had six patients who fit this profile? Would your workload for that shift be easier or harder? Most definitely, it would be harder.

Next, a mean nurse will sometimes harp at you to discharge a patient when you're in the middle of something. For instance, you just got a new patient and the doctor wants an IV started right away so IV antibiotics can be given. In walks the mean nurse, who informs you that another patient of yours is up for discharge. But, here's the kicker—the mean nurse knows that a patient needing immediate IV antibiotics takes priority over a stable patient who's ready to be discharged home.

Another way nurses are singled out is by getting a new admit even though it's not their turn. Maybe they took the last admit, or the one before that, and there are nurses who haven't had a new admit yet. One day while working in the ER I got assigned an ambulance patient – no big deal, but that made four patients for me while the other two nurses (whom I had stood up to recently) had three patients *total* between the two of them. Needless to say, while I never heard the clash of forks and knives, I definitely felt like I was on the menu for lunch that day.

In addition to these types of behaviors, mean nurses will also lie about you, hoping to rally others, for they have an exaggerated sense of self and want to be in control of all aspects of the work environment. This includes how you take care of your patients, your happiness at work, and what others think of you.

So what's a nice nurse – or just a neutral, hardworking nurse – to do? From my experience you have two options: First option, you acknowledge that life isn't fair and you face this mean nonsense with as much grace and dignity that you can possibly muster. Second option, you fight, hold your ground, point out the examples of unfairness, and even run to HR if you feel you must.

I'll tell you which option from my experience I think is best, and that is option number one. Keep a cool head, and if you're not currently in possession of grace and dignity, find some! Here's why: Nurses working in the same department must work as a team. In most hospital departments, nurses are assigned their own patients, but circumstances often arise that force nurses to depend on each other.

For example: When I worked in the ER I had patients in critical condition that needed a CT scan, which was located down the hall in radiology. But, when patients are unstable the nurse must accompany them while the CT scan is being done. At the same time, I had other patients in the ER, and therefore another nurse had to look out for them while I was gone. He had his own assigned patients but also had to cover mine, and I did the same for him when he had to accompany a critical patient to radiology.

Here's another example: Let's say you're working on a medical/ surgical floor and you have six patients. You're informed at the same time that one of your patients is having severe chest pain and another patient just vomited blood everywhere. How do you decide which patient to see first? You don't! Both of these situations are critical and both demand a nurse's attention. So you're left with one option: you see one of your patients and you *ask* another nurse to check on the other one.

Now, imagine that the nurse you need to ask for help is one you've went to war with. First off, it's likely to be uncomfortable asking for their help. Secondly, in the back of your mind you're going to wonder if they really will take care of your patient. And lastly, some of them will tell you no, making some excuse about doing something for one of their own patients.

And in case you're thinking, *Surely there'll be a nice nurse around to ask for help,* well, sometimes yes and sometimes no. They might be down the hall passing meds, or starting an IV, or in the cafeteria grabbing lunch. At times, your only option is to ask a mean nurse for help.

Can a mean nurse make excuses or refuse to help even if you don't go to war with them? Absolutely, but it's less likely. From my experience, when you remain kind and professional towards a mean nurse and sincerely ask for help, it's hard for them to say no. Go to war with them, and you'll find it's a different story.

Does the concept of nurses eating their young mainly apply to new nurses? It can, but not necessarily. I've seen nurses of all ages and experience levels deal with this. The main difference is because older nurses have usually endured more trials, they know how to get a handle on these situations more easily.

If you choose NOT to become a nurse, will you likely face someone who's mean in a different career? Yes, but in the medical profession the stakes are higher because someone's life or well-being is on the line. In some occupations, if you have a disagreement with someone you can walk away and take ten; as a nurse you don't usually have this option. And, yes, there are other jobs where people are required to work together and it'd be frustrating if someone didn't pull their fair share; but, again, not the same as a patient possibly losing their life with a follow-up investigation of, *What went wrong with the nurses who couldn't suck it up and work together?*

Are ALL nurses mean? No, but there's certainly enough of them that I'd dare to venture they have their own secret club. I've never been invited.

Is nurses eating their young a concept that mainly applies to hospital nursing? Absolutely. If you work for a home health or hospice company, you have your assigned patients and see them one at a time. Or if you work in a physician's office, as a school nurse, or for an insurance company, most of your work is done independently. Not all nurses work for hospitals; although, it's a great place to build up your experience and skills before moving into other nursing positions.

The majority of my own nursing career has played out within the confines of hospitals, and I'll admit to not always handling mean nurses in the best possible way. Many times when targeted by a mean nurse I became withdrawn, downtrodden, or I desperately wanted to tell everyone my side, and sometimes did.

After some experience my advice now is this – don't do ANY of these. If there's a situation between you and a mean nurse that's constantly affecting patient care and could yield negative patient outcomes, then you have an ethical obligation to address it. Otherwise, keep smiling, remain engaged with others, and support your fellow nurses. People are far more intuitive than we give them credit for; eventually, they figure out the truth all on their own.

CHAPTER 13

Be prepared to walk a tightrope with physicians.

Many years ago when working on a medical/surgical floor, a physician at the start of my 7 a.m. shift started venting (at me) because a nurse on nightshift didn't handle his patient correctly. He proceeded to tell me what the nurse didn't do, what she should've done, and the consequence to the patient.

All the while I was thinking, *You've got to be kidding me!* After all, I wasn't the nurse who messed up, and I had multiple patients to see, meds to pass, assessments to complete – and this moron was being inconsiderate and wasting my time!

Did I express this to the physician? Of course not! Instead, I didn't dare take my eyes off of him, I listened intently to his ranting, I nodded in agreement when appropriate, and no doubt at some point uttered the words, *Yes, sir.*

Why? Because working with physicians* is complicated. No, they're not our direct bosses (they don't do our yearly evaluation or write us up if we're tardy), but they do initiate the orders, procedures, etc., that we as nurses follow. Therefore, we're in contact with physicians frequently, and it's like unto a symbiotic relationship. Physicians need nurses to carry out orders, and nurses need physicians to provide those orders.

Simply put – whether you work for a hospital, clinic, physician's office, home health, or hospice company – as nurses, we need them to do our job. Even though physicians write most of their own orders, nurses often approach physicians with a concern or question that a patient has, or to report a critical lab value, or to ask for new medication orders, etc. And, yes, physicians are highly educated and usually professional, but they are still affected by human emotions the same as anyone else. If a nurse is on good terms with a physician, it's going to be much easier to approach them and get what you need to do your job and take care of your patient. If you're not on good terms, the opposite will be true as well.

In regards to other careers, approaching a fellow coworker for advice, or referencing a past project or file, or just finding creative ways to solve work-related obstacles are perfectly acceptable. In nursing, it's OK to ask other nurses for help if you haven't done something before, *but you've got to know what your exact orders are and they COME from physicians.*

Is every encounter I have with physicians like the one referenced above? No, but there's certainly been enough of them that I consider myself "schooled" in this area. So without delay, here are my tips (acquired through much grief and agony) for working with physicians.

Give them their due. Physicians work hard to get where they're at so — regardless of whether you like them or not, or whether they're a seasoned physician or one who's brand new — address them appropriately and be respectful.

Be mindful of their personality and demeanor. Are they easygoing, matter-of-fact, somewhere in the middle? Approach them accordingly.

Get to the point and take notes. When you approach a physician, know exactly what you're going to ask for or inform them about. If you need to go over several things, write them down and write down the physician's responses. It's easy to get sidetracked, but quite humiliating to later repeat these conversations while they stare at you like you belong in the zoo.

Always catch the physician in person if you can. Physicians get frustrated if they're making rounds and accessible and then you page them as they're driving home or having dinner with their family. Also, there are physicians with practices located away from the hospital; therefore, they come in early, during lunch, or after their practice is closed to see patients who are admitted under their care.

I once worked with a physician in this situation. He would arrive at the hospital early and then go to his primary practice. At the time, I was still learning the rhythm of getting my assessments done and was preoccupied with not getting behind. So I would get what I needed done first and then page him to address what I needed on his patients. One day he said to me on the phone, "Nancy, I'm not getting on to you, but please try to address these things with me while I'm on the floor. Then if anything comes up during the day, feel free to page me. But I'm NOT getting on to you." For months I'd been inconveniencing this kind physician, and I didn't have a clue.

Use the word 'clarify' when possible. Physicians have a lot on their plate, so sometimes they write orders that aren't completely clear. For example, a physician writes an order for 'dressing changes to the right ankle twice daily.' But, you're not sure what type of dressing change the physician wants. So you approach or call the physician and say something like, "I just wanted to clarify regarding your order for dressing changes on this patient. Do you want a basic wet-to-dry dressing, or was there something else you had in mind?"

By approaching physicians and clarifying orders, you won't come across as criticizing them for not writing a clear order; and you're showing them you care enough about the patient and doing what the physician wants to follow up on the order.

Anticipate follow-up questions and have those answers

ready. If you page a physician to inform them their patient's blood pressure was elevated at 2 p.m., they're more than likely going to ask you what the previous two blood pressures were. They'll want to know if it has been trending up all day or if this was the first occurrence.

When absolutely necessary, stand your ground with a physician. First, if they ever tell you to do something outside your scope of practice, don't do it. Next, we all have times when we just can't take it anymore, but pick your battles wisely and fight them with the least amount of ammunition necessary.

For example, I once had a patient whom the physician had discussed going home with home health or possibly going to a skilled nursing facility. Now, there are different things needing to be done for either one of those to happen, and I knew the patient's discharge date was near. So I approached the physician, but as soon as he saw me he said, "I don't have time for a lengthy conversation with you."

This physician had pushed my buttons one too many times and I'd had enough, so I locked eyes with him and frankly replied, "Nor do I wish to have a lengthy conversation with *you.*"

Our battle was quick but enough of one to get his attention, and then afterwards we quickly discussed what was necessary for both of us to do our jobs and moved on.

Now in complete fairness to physicians we must consider this: Physicians have a tremendous amount of responsibility. They're admitting new patients, seeing existing patients, reviewing labs on everyone, deciding which tests to order, changing medications, dictating progress notes, and consulting any needed specialists. They work long hours, usually have insane student loans to repay, and don't see their families as often as they'd like; so they don't always intend to be snappy or short or unclear about what you need to do. No doubt, they're doing the best they can.

Lastly, no matter how good *your* intentions are, sometimes things just won't go as planned. I experienced such a moment when I went to work in the NICU (Newborn Intensive Care Unit). My preceptor introduced me to a particular doctor one morning and it went like this: "Dr. So-and-so (name withheld of course), this is Nancy; she's a new RN and will be working the nightshift."

Now, during this time I was young, excited, and eager to meet all the players. So I smiled brightly, thrust my hand forward to shake, and said, "Hello!"

It became clear my enthusiasm wouldn't be reciprocated when the physician looked me up and down, then slightly tilted her head and said, "Hum."

---

*physicians, physician assistants and/or nurse practitioners; anyone directing patient care that a nurse would report to, and receive orders from.

CHAPTER 14

The family wants me to do what?

I once encountered a family member who wanted their loved one's admit status to be changed from observation to a full admit. The family knew that if the patient was officially admitted and stayed three full nights in the hospital, then they would've qualified for skilled services in a nursing home under Medicare. However, the patient's admitting diagnosis and criteria didn't qualify them for full admit status; therefore, they were in the hospital as observation. The family wanted us (me and/or the physician) to change the patient to a full admit to obtain the skilled services.

As graciously as possible, this Oklahoma nurse tried to explain that if we changed the patient to a full admit – knowing they didn't meet medical guidelines for that status – it could result in Medicare fraud for the hospital. My legal concerns *and* restraints appeared to have fallen on deaf ears, for the patient's daughter simply replied, "You know nothing."

This was a disappointing moment for me as I truly wanted to help the patient as much as I could; but, this hasn't been the only frustrating encounter I've had with family members. I've also been confronted by families demanding a particular test be done even though it's unrelated to what the patient was admitted for, such as an MRI of the brain on granny when she's in the hospital for pneumonia. Or requesting a loved one be given IV fluids because they appear dehydrated. Never mind that the patient is in kidney failure – the family knows what they need.

And here's an example I've experienced many times working in a clinic: Parents keep their kids out of school all week because they're sick but don't bring them in to be seen until Thursday or Friday, and now they want a note for school covering the entire week's absence.

Often during these times, if you don't carry out what the families want, they'll imply you're stupid or that you don't want to help, not knowing or caring that you need a physician's order or approval for most of their requests. And sometimes they'll conjure up stories and rationales to support what they want, like, *My cousin went through this exact same thing two years ago in Dallas and they did it for him.* If you still don't comply, they'll threaten to report you to your superior. I've often provided directions to the administration office.

Nevertheless, in the medical field there are standards of care that must be upheld, which include having appropriate orders, testing based on the current diagnosis and symptoms, medication and IV administration based on clinical data, and providing work and/or school notes cor-relating with when a patient was actually seen and treated by a medical provider.

Now, if it's possible the issues with family are just a case of confusion or misunderstanding, I recommend pa-tience and education. Try to explain that if the doctor or-ders a test unrelated to the patient's diagnosis and current needs the insurance company may not cover it, and discuss the need for hydration in relation to kidney function.

However, if the family pushes you to do something unethical, I recommend addressing it immediately. And, if there's a policy, procedure guide, or standard of care where you work to fall back on – do it! This doesn't ease the tension with all family members, but it will help with some.

Being in a position to receive requests or demands from family members can happen in *almost* any area of nursing practice but tends to occur more frequently re-garding patients who are younger or older. As a matter of fact, my mom and I took my grandma to an appointment with her orthopedist one day. As we were heading out the door of the nursing home, a staff member requested all orders be faxed in addition to us bringing them back with us. So what did I do? I passed this request onto the ortho-pedist's nurse, even though it seemed redundant to fax then hand deliver the orders when we returned grandma.

Sometimes the requests families make are legitimate

and we should do our best to accommodate them; other times they are not, resulting in wasted time nurses don't have and argumentative conversations that actually misdirect the nurse's time *away* from patient care.

Lastly, while some families are sincere and forthcoming, don't be afraid to ask questions if something seems off. A physician and I once encountered a patient's loved one who insisted we order some particular tests, all the while telling us she was a doctor. The physician was very patient and tried to explain what tests could be ordered in relation to the patient's diagnosis and symptoms.

At last, with no reprieve, the physician began asking questions of her own, and what she discovered was remarkable. The patient's loved one was indeed a doctor, but one of veterinary medicine.

Staying Legal and Keeping Your License

CHAPTER 15

Nurses are NOT puppets, so be prepared
to think and act for yourself.

I heard through the grapevine long ago that an extended family member of mine had said, "All nurses do is pass pills." Had this been true, and had I known it, I would've jumped on this gravy train much sooner. I also couldn't help but look around and wonder where all the Chimpanzees were. If they can indeed be trained to do just about anything, why not pass pills and temper the nationwide nursing shortage?

In addition to only passing pills, it's also been speculated that nurses just follow orders. The physician gives the orders, and the obedient nurse completes them. Now, this is true but only to a certain point. In chapter 13 I stressed the importance of effective communication with physicians in order to obtain all needed orders. But here's the 4-1-1 on this: Nurses are responsible for ALL orders – including those that are wrong or contraindicated – if they're CARRIED out. Therefore, even when we are CLEAR on what the physician wants, we still must check and make sure the orders are appropriate for our patient. We also must use our skills and training as nurses to know when to interrupt, or stop, an order.

For example: A physician gives an order for a patient to have blood pressure medicine every morning at 9 a.m., but the patient's blood pressure at that time is on the low side at 80/50. *What do you do?* You hold the medication and notify the physician of the patient's blood pressure.

Here's another example: You have an order to give 15mg of morphine via IV for pain. As a skilled nurse, you realize that's an extremely high dose. *What do you do?* First, check and see how much morphine the patient's been receiving. If you find they've been getting 5mg IV, question the physician about the order, because here's the reality: If you carry out this order 'as is' and the patient goes into respiratory depression from too much morphine, it's on YOUR license, not the physician's.

If a doctor orders an antibiotic and you find it on your patient's list of allergies, politely inform the doctor and see what other antibiotic they want. Not familiar with a medication ordered? Don't give it! Reference a drug book first and learn the correct dosage, route, side effects, and counter-indications. If the drug book doesn't yield sufficient information, check with a pharmacist.

Another skill you must acquire as a nurse is being proactive on behalf of your patients. Let's say you have a patient who falls and hits her head. There's no bleeding and the patient didn't lose consciousness. *What do you do?* You call, page, or chase the physician down, if necessary, and report this.

Subsequently, if the physician gives you an order, such as "send the patient to radiology for a CT of the head," you do it and then document everything. But let's say you tell the physician and they don't give you any orders. *What do you do?* You document, 'Notified physician X that at 11:05 patient Y fell and hit her head. No orders were received from physician X at this time.'

By documenting that you notified the physician of the incident and NO orders were received, if the patient develops a head bleed due to the fall and slips into a coma, YOU won't be liable for it because you did everything you could at that time within your scope as a nurse. Now, if the patient develops slurred speech two hours later, you must go back to the physician and start the process over.

Why so much fuss about checking orders, asking questions, and being proactive? Here's why: If you do NOT step up and take action on behalf of your patient when you should, or you DO something (even unintentionally) that causes adverse harm to a patient – that according to standard nursing practice a trained nurse should know NOT to do – you could lose your license and/or be sued for malpractice.

This necessity for nurses to be on their toes applies to *any* nursing position that involves patient care. If you work as a home health nurse and discover during your visit that your patient's heart rate is elevated and he's running a fever, you would notify the physician overseeing his care and anticipate orders. Or, what if you work for a family medicine physician and while administering a routine flu shot the patient started having difficulty breathing? You would immediately have someone go get the physician, even if they were in another room with a patient.

Being a nurse isn't a job you can take lightly or put on autopilot; we are responsible for countless lives. We don't just pass pills, nor do we sit around waiting for the almighty physician to hand us our marching orders. So I'll say this one last time: think, ask questions, examine every order and be proactive when needed. Physicians may chart the course for patient care, but nurses are front and center.

CHAPTER 16

If you don't chart it – you didn't do it,
see it, and it didn't happen!

One day while saturated with charting and patient care I received a phone call. The voice on the other end informed me that several years prior I'd taken care of a woman in the ER who had been assaulted. At some point she'd filed charges against her husband; he was fighting them in court and I was on the list as a potential witness. I was told that in situations like this the judge would occasionally allow the nurse's charting to be read aloud in court, without the nurse testifying on the stand. I received an official subpoena just in case.

As I set the receiver down I searched for this woman in the depths of my memory but could not find her, and it broke my heart. If I couldn't remember her face, her name, or that I even treated her – how could I have possibly charted enough to save her when she needed me the most?

Approximately two weeks later I met with someone from the legal team at the hospital. The court date was drawing near and I was to remain on standby. In preparation for what might lie ahead, I asked if I could review the patient's medical records. In most cases, once a patient is discharged from a facility you don't access their records again unless medically necessary. An exception was made and I was given her information.

Later, alone, on a computer away from others I entered her name and date of birth. As I came across the skin assessment and saw my documentation of bruise after bruise, size and locations, floodgates of relief washed over me. The dreaded day eventually came and I was not required to testify; my documentation was *more* than sufficient.

As nurses, and regardless of which setting we practice in, we have a window of opportunity to chart what we need to. In some circumstances, we *can* later document something we forgot but the chart will reflect that, and if it's reviewed in court you will be heavily questioned regarding the time lapse. Therefore, it's in the best interest of nurses to chart everything we need to in the moment. In addition to all cases of abuse and neglect, here are some other occurrences you'd definitely want to chart.

If a patient arrives to your facility from a nursing home with an indwelling urinary catheter in place, you'd chart that. Why? Indwelling urinary catheters need to be changed from time to time and are known for causing horrific infections. Oftentimes, when a patient arrives with one in place it will be removed and replaced with a new one. But, if the patient develops a horrible urinary infection and you do NOT document that they arrived with a urinary catheter in place, the facility could be blamed for the infection, when in fact it was caused by the urinary catheter they *arrived* with and not the new one that you placed.

Also, there are some IV medications that are known for being hard on the veins; they infuse slower than other medications and require a watchful eye. If you have a situation like this, you'd want to check on the IV frequently and chart you did so every time. *Can something start to go wrong with an IV minutes after walking away from it?* Yes, but if you've been documenting at regular intervals that you checked it, it will help affirm that any complication was a mere coincidence and not due to your neglect.

In this profession there are countless examples of situations that should be charted, but in wrapping up, here's my last one: In many ERs and clinics, if a patient receives an antibiotic shot, they are required to wait for a certain length of time before they can leave (usually 15-30 minutes). Some patients, unknown to them at the time, are allergic to antibiotics. If they are going to have an allergic reaction, it will usually occur within that time frame, and with them NOT yet being discharged, you can jump in and give the needed medications to counter this reaction. However, it is possible that a patient could have a reaction after the required wait time. To cover yourself, show that you're adhering to policy and abiding by the medical standard of care by documenting, *Antibiotic wait hold complete, no signs or symptoms of reaction noted, patient discharged home.* Or something close to it!

CHAPTER 17

You may feel like you're crashing,
but don't abandon your patients.

My eyes wouldn't stop searching for the clock. I didn't want them to; it felt wrong and yet my efforts to turn their gaze fell flat. *Was I a fraud?* Aren't nurses supposed to be tough, resilient, compassionate? Able to respond, adapt, handle anything – for any length of time? But I just wanted out. There'd been an endless stream of critical patients in the ER all day, and I was slipping beneath the surface fast.

When I finally heard the night shift crew filter in, I exhaled. I could give report to my replacement, walk away with my dignity intact, and then drive off as fast as possible. So I put on a brave face for my patients and myself, believing that my rescue was imminent – yet no one came for me. After what felt like forever the night charge nurse came into view and told me my replacement was running late. "You can give report and leave when she gets here," she said bluntly.

As she turned her back to me and walked away, a series of events unfolded: It started as pressure in my chest that quickly rose to my head – my blood pressure had just spiked. Next, my hands and arms became numb, started tingling, and I felt dizzy. The last symptom to hit was blurry vision. How on earth would I be able to take care of my patients when I could barely see? But no one came for me, and I couldn't leave.

Had I came in off the street as a patient and checked in with these symptoms, I would've been attended to. But in all honesty, this wasn't a medical issue; it was a nurse issue. I'd worked 12-plus hours with no break, barely a chance to pee, and hardly any food. My nervous system was shot and I was on the brink. *What did I do?* The only thing I could. I hung on until the consistently late nightshift nurse showed up.

If you're considering this profession and think, *I can handle any type of patient or working environment or chaos, as long as I'm out when my time's up!* then know this: Things don't always go as planned. Your co-workers WILL call in, they WILL run late, you WILL get hit with multiple admits or a code blue at the most inconvenient time. And staying beyond your time or limits is not just applicable to hospital nursing. If you work as a home health nurse and arrive to find your patient has taken a turn for the worse and is medically unstable, you can't leave. If you work in a clinic and someone checks in right at closing time, you're staying.

What happens if you leave your patient when they're medically unstable or when the charge nurse has specifically told you not to? You could be charged with patient abandonment. Physicians and paramedics can also be charged with patient abandonment, but let's look at how this applies to nurses.

According to the Oklahoma Board of Nursing, found online at ok.gov, the definition is this: "Abandonment may occur when a licensed nurse fails to provide adequate patient care until the responsibility for care of the patient is assumed by another licensed nurse or an approved licensed health care provider. Patient safety is the key factor in determining the nurse's responsibility in a given situation."

Also listed on the website are additional guidelines and specific situations that may constitute abandonment.

My advice to you is this: Look up your state nursing website and carefully review the patient abandonment law and any additional guidelines or specific situations. Next, go into this profession expecting these situations to happen from time to time. Finally, be prepared (as much as you can) for the unexpected.

For many years I carried several bite-sized Snicker candy bars in my pockets when I worked in the ER; never knowing if I'd have time to eat an actual meal. One day I bent over to pick something up and out they fell. A little blonde-headed girl I was taking care of pointed, giggled, and said in a singsong voice, "Your candy fell out of your pocket."

Well, yes it did, but it was sealed in a wrapper and at least I got to eat something… that shift.

CHAPTER 18

Shhh, you can't share that!

A while back I had quite an interesting experience in a mall bathroom. I entered the stall and was in position to do my business when I overheard a girl on her cell a few stalls down from me. Now, I hadn't intended to eavesdrop, but once I picked up the thread of conversation I didn't know what to do. If I proceeded with my intentions she might discover my presence and stop talking, or worse, if she had violent tendencies. After brief contemplation, I decided to remain incognito until she vacated the premises.

When I was finally able to get down to business, I found myself shocked by her candid conversation but then questioned why I would be. After all, we thrive in a culture of sharing and not much is off limits. We share date night, what we eat, where we go, how we feel, and just about everything else we can think of. As a matter of fact, a while back I cut my finger chopping onions. *What did I do?* I reached for my phone and posted it to Facebook, of course – all the while dripping blood on my kitchen counter. Don't fret, I have bleach.

While sharing moments like these between friends can indeed be entertaining, if you become a nurse you'd better learn to keep a lid on it when it comes to patient information. For many years there were no laws or regulations addressing this, but in 1996, HIPAA (Health Insurance Portability and Accountability Act) was established. This helps govern medical facilities (hospitals, home health companies, doctor's offices, etc.) as well as individuals who work at these facilities and have access to medical records.

In a nutshell, patients have the right to protect identifiable health information about themselves, and when medical entities do share information, it must be in a confidential and secure manner. This does not interfere with normal business procedures, such as submitting a claim with a patient's insurance. This is in regard to a business sharing information with another party when it's not necessary, in an unsecure way, or an *individual* sharing or accessing medical information NOT needed to do their job.

Now, I don't want to drown you in legal phrases and terminology, but I do want to offer some practical examples of HIPAA violations.

Example #1 – A hospice nurse has just left her patient's home when a sweet neighbor approaches her car and motions to roll down the window. She then proceeds to ask with much sincerity if the patient's cancer has finally become terminal. The hospice nurse confirms the neighbor's suspicions.

This is a HIPAA violation. Yes, obviously the neighbor already had knowledge of the patient's diagnosis of cancer, but the nurse had no authority to confirm that it was terminal or comment in any way about her medical condition.

Example #2 – A nurse is working in the ER when in walks the prom king from high school, escorted by a police officer. He was picked up for public intoxication, but he also has a laceration that's actively bleeding, and they need him stitched up before he heads off to the can. The ER nurse begins to text about the downfall of prince charming to her friends.

This is a HIPAA violation. The nurse has no right to share anything about the patient's visit. Even if the prom king sought treatment for a sore throat after a night of karaoke, it would still be a violation if shared.

Example #3 – A school nurse is out grocery shopping when approached by a longtime friend. Her friend mentions by name a high school senior who's pregnant and asks if she knows what the student has decided to do with the baby. The school nurse reveals that the student is considering placing the baby with an adoption service.

This is a HIPAA violation. It doesn't matter that the nurse's friend knew the student by name, and it doesn't matter if the student is far enough along that the entire community can tell she's pregnant – any information the nurse has acquired about the student's plans is confidential and protected.

I think these examples are fairly clear, but nurses can also violate HIPAA in less obvious ways. If a nurse goes into a patient's room to do an assessment (be it a room in a hospital or a home health visit) and the patient has visitors, the nurse needs to look at the patient and say something along the lines of, *I need to ask you a lot of questions so I can best take care of you. Is it OK to ask questions in front of your visitors?* This way, the nurse has asked permission and it's up to the patient whether to share his/her information.

Also, in regard to hospitals, nursing homes, and rehabilitation facilities, visitors will sometimes come to the nurses' desk and ask questions about patients. Nurses must be on guard about this. Some visitors have been given permission by the patient to do this, while others have not. An honest mistake can still be a HIPAA violation.

Another frequent occurrence is this: You're taking care of a patient in one of the above mentioned settings when one of *their* visitors walks in and says, *I just passed my good friend Johnny in a wheelchair. What's he in for?* At this time you look at the visitor and say, *I'm sorry, but I can't discuss anyone's medical information with you; it's against the law.*

Keep in mind that most people are just curious and conversational. They're not trying to get you in trouble, but you still need to protect your patients and yourself.

So what happens if a person or facility is charged with a HIPAA violation? According to the American Medical Association, found online, "Failure to comply with HIPAA can result in civil and criminal penalties, including up to 10 years in prison and up to $250,000 in fines for facilities or individuals."

Finally, be wary of everyone. Two coworkers and I were in the breakroom one day when in came a lady wearing a suit with an employee badge turned around. My coworkers and I didn't know who she was and carried on eating lunch. After a few minutes one of my companions started talking about a difficult patient, referencing her by name.

I, being a play-by-the-books-kind-of-girl, didn't say a word but noticed the unknown female looking restless. At last she revealed why when she blurted out, "Guys, I'm the HIPAA officer for this facility!"

Come to find out, she was there to discuss HIPAA compliancy with as many available employees as possible and was just waiting for the manager to round up some more. Obviously, she'd come to the right department.

Final Thoughts…

I've found that some enroll in nursing school already knowing what they want. They want to work a day shift, at a doctor's office, for the health department, or only with babies so there's no heavy lifting. Well, kudos to them and possibly you for thinking ahead, but keep in mind that whatever you want others will want too, and you may not land where you want starting off. Just keep your chin up, accept the next best offer at the time, and fight for your place.

The other side of this is that after you've been a nurse for a reasonable amount of time, prospective employers will target YOU. Currently, about twice a month I receive a phone call or something by mail with a job offer, or a solicitation to inquire about a position I have experience in. This is all well and good and a great reminder of the job security in this field, but you and I would be wise to remember the saying about that grass on the other side of the fence. I've NEVER worked in a nursing position where absolutely everything was perfect. Although, if you become a nurse and discover glistening greener pastures, I do hope you'll feel compelled to share them with me.

On a different note I'll say this: My time as a nurse has taught me to think on my feet, be bold, and adapt on the fly. I've learned to give more when I was certain I was empty. I've made friendships I'll never forget and laugh when I reminisce about the messes I've got into, and out of. Like the time I put a wet washcloth in the microwave; my plan was to put it on my forehead to ease my headache. Unfortunately, I left it in too long, it caught on fire, I had to try to get rid of the smoke *before* the doctor came in for his morning rounds – and I still had a throbbing headache!

I can't guarantee that you or others will create memories like these, or that being a nurse will change you for the better or be the *right* career for you. As for me, being a nurse has helped make me stronger, kinder, and more resourceful – and I wouldn't trade those attributes for anything.

Lastly, I've done my absolute best to provide you with the essential pieces of this profession. However, after reading this if you have a particular question or concern that's hindering you from making a decision, feel free to contact me and I'll do my best to assist you with your (career selection) issues.

Here's wishing you all the best on your journey, whatever you choose it to be.

Nurse Nancy